Brain Rejuvenation

Regan Archibald, Lac, FMP, CSSAc

Here's What's Inside...

A Story about Your Brain

In my teen years, I would ride my Honda racing motorcycle across the St. Anthony Sand Dunes in Idaho. One summer afternoon, at the end of a long day of riding, I was struck by another rider and knocked out. My motionless arm sizzled on my exhaust pipe until my friend was able to pull the bike off me. When I finally woke up, the feeling of disorientation and the stabbing headache made me want to sleep again. When I arrived at the hospital, my arm had third-degree burns, but the doctors were most concerned about my brain. They kept a close watch, and soon released me without any treatment beyond some anti-inflammatory prescriptions.

It took several months before I felt like myself. I had a great support team with my mother leading the cause, but even with all the love they showed me, I didn't feel like myself. I noticed episodes of depression and social anxiety. I didn't sleep well and suffered from insomnia until my mid-thirties. Luckily, I was able to keep my grades high enough not to cause any concern, but I lost interest in the subjects that had most interested me and even lost interest in hanging out with friends. This was certainly the most severe of several traumatic brain injuries that I've experienced throughout my life; looking back, if I had the knowledge then that I do now, I could have successfully treated my brain and enjoyed my teenage years much more. It's not that I wasn't proactive; I read books and articles on memory and brain health, and even bought a program called Mega Memory to see if I could regain what was lost. All of this was helpful, but I can't imagine the amount of difference that stem cell therapy would have made for my young, developing brain.

Shortly after my accident, the importance of brain health was further driven home when I noticed that my grandmother's memory was slipping. She was an inspiring woman who had nothing but vitality and enthusiasm for life. She had raised five kids and was heavily involved in community events, but she lost it all to Alzheimer's disease. Her bright eyes became dull and full of confusion. She would burst into fits of frustration and rage that no amount of reasoning could calm. Her health independence was lost at an early age; though she had lived a great life, she died a miserable death, riddled with complications of one of the deadliest brain diseases that I wouldn't wish on my worst enemy.

Perhaps you've picked up this book because you are either looking for ways to reverse brain disease or prevent it for yourself or a loved one. I believe that if I can inspire even one person to commit to treating their brain and regaining their health independence, then this book will be worth the effort of writing it.

Enjoy the book!

Your brain is at the very core of your experience of being human; this small organ dictates your quality of life, your capabilities, and even controls your emotions. Your brain is a three-pound organ that can conjure brilliance, mastery, happiness, and even heartbreak. It is your portal to the past, and the gateway to your future. It provides you with dreams and nightmares, breakthroughs and debilitating anxiety. It's time to give your brain some love.

The brilliance of this organ cannot be overstated. Think of every scientific discovery that has been made, every single problem that has been solved, and every bit of creative artistry that has ever been dreamt up—all of this wonder is the product of one specific organ that comes standard with each human being. Your brain has uniquely evolved over the past four million years to become capable of genius creations, ideas, and thoughts.

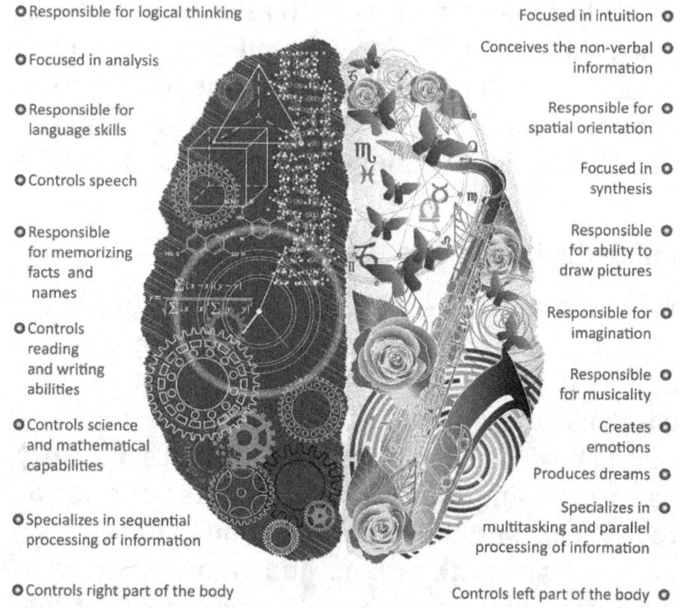

But most likely, you've been taught that your fragile brain, once damaged, can't heal. Even some of the most damaged brains can heal from serious diseases like Alzheimer's, Parkinson 's disease, or even depression.

You will see that brains that have endured concussions, strokes, or Post-Traumatic Stress Disorder (PTSD) can all recover with breakthrough treatments using medicinal signaling stem cells that safely and easily access the most damaged parts of your brain and work at healing it.

Your brain is arguably the most important component of your body. I now love my brain, and the more I have learned to work with it, the happier I have become.

Treating my brain has been the best investment in my health that I could have made. Because of my new brain health, I look forward to aging chronologically, because I've learned some things that can keep my biology young.

Because of my brain health, I have been able to build up a very successful integrated medical practice that now has four clinics in Utah called East West Health. I have authored four different books, created 15 different medical training programs, and am a frequent speaker with my Go Wellness practitioners.

I have also founded the Stem Cell Health Centers, which is a network of practices using breakthrough brain treatments. I am a lucky husband and the father of the most amazing kids on the planet!

My mission is to end brain disease and pain for a million people over the next seven years. None of this would be possible if I weren't able to find ways to repair the damage that was inflicted on my brain.

I hope to provide you with the answers you are looking for so that you can keep and reclaim your brain health, and have .brain rejuvenation through the rest of your life.

Most people become aware of their brain at the point when it no longer works properly.

To better brain health!

Regan

Preventing Brain Degeneration – Is It Possible?

Only when your brain isn't operating at the level to which you are accustomed, do you start to realize the necessity of a healthy brain. You try to get your brain engaged in a new thought process. You search unsuccessfully to find the name of that individual who you've met a million times. You wonder where you left your keys, to no avail. These moments when our brains appear to misfire may happen daily. At these times, you may curse your brain for its inability and disorganized filing system. Our brains can frustrate us to no end, as we wonder why they will not work efficiently!

The problem is that we only become aware of the brain when it is not firing on all cylinders. As we get older, these glitches become more and more frequent. We berate this phenomenal organ and lament that it is not serving us as we believe it should. If only we had given this kind of consideration to our brains back when they were was working efficiently. When brain degeneration happens, we experience a significant drop in brain performance; in some cases, the degeneration leads to more chronic diseases that most doctors will blame on age. My goal is to show you a new path with stem cell therapy that has the potential to be a safe, effective, and easy way to regenerate your brain and make it new again.

The truth is, the brain is one of the most under acknowledged organs in our entire body until it stops working effectively. Once it stops working, there are novel ways of turning it back on, regardless of what your diagnosis may be.

How is your brain performing at a level of 1 to 10, with ten being ideal and 0 being non-functional? At what level would you like it to operate?

What are the major obstacles/diseases that are getting in your way of having a dynamic, healthy brain?

Regenerate Your Brain

What if I proposed a way for you to regenerate your brain? Rather than sit in the audience watching in frustration as your brain performance deteriorates, you can take active steps toward ensuring that this show goes on in all its glory. Imagine that you could look after your brain in the same way you look after the rest of your body. Now there is a concrete way to show appreciation for this vital organ before it is too late.

Have you ever suffered the disorientating effects of a concussion? Perhaps you had a bicycle accident as a child, or fell down the stairs, or suffered a blow during a football game? Maybe you have been through an unthinkable event in your life that has brought on Post-Traumatic Stress Disorder. These are some of the unfortunate events and accidents that can contribute to brain degeneration.

The distressing part is the idea that our brains can't regenerate themselves. We've been told that once you lose brain cells, they're gone for good. This is a rather alarming thought. How could an accident in my teenage years, or my response to a terrifying event, irreversibly impact my capacity to think, process, and remember? Can it be that with all of our technological advancements, we are still at the mercy of a slap in the face by fate?

I am here to tell you that it doesn't have to be this way. Imagine that you could have brain rejuvenation throughout your entire life. Imagine yourself not having to be at the mercy of circumstance, accident, and aging. Imagine that you could increase the amount of time with this precious organ operating at optimum capacity. Imagine that your agency determined how well your brain would work as you move forward in life.

The good news is that you no longer have to imagine. The optimal, ongoing use of your brain right into your later years is now possible, through a process of brain regeneration.

I am going to guide you through some of the most enthralling research about this magnificent part of the human body. By showing you how to increase and improve the longevity and health of your brain, I hope to turn any possible feelings of defeat you may have into optimism and clarity for your future health. You will start to see that you will not only be able to retain your current cognitive functioning, but improve on it.

Many of the studies that have allowed me to write this book and create the brain regeneration protocols can be found at **www.stemcellhealthcenters.com** or **www.acueastwest.com**. I hope that this will translate into you having a long-term relationship with your own healthy, productive brain.

Sounds Interesting, But How?

At this point, I am sure that your brain's receptors have perked up and a big, red HOW? Sign is flashing at your brain's epicenter. It may sound wonderful in theory, but can I rejuvenate my brain to live a productive and happy life? How does this work in reality?

This very question is at the core of our mission at East West Health. We work towards ensuring that you improve and maintain your health for the longest time possible. One of my greatest missions in life is to make and enhance brain health for every single patient. While we offer various treatments to optimize health, this book focuses on one in particular—*ending brain deterioration with perinatal tissue therapy.*

You may be thinking, "Now you have lost me," and this may be a challenging concept to digest at first. One idea, hammered into us from a very young age, is that aging (and its companion, deterioration) is completely inevitable; we cannot do anything to slow or reverse these processes. And stem cells? Aren't those the things used to clone people with?

I'm here to tell you that the deterioration of your brain is by no means inevitable: There is a way for you to keep your brain functioning at an optimal level well into your final years. As for stem cells, well, you are on the right track. The perinatal tissue is used for creation and rejuvenation, but this is not limited to a Frankenstein-like conjuring of new human life. The growth factors, cytokines, and stem cells can change the course of your journey in the direction of optimal wellness.

If you decide to go on this journey with me, you will find that the purposes for which stem cells can be used are far more varied and intricate than you may have previously thought. Through a combination of modern scientific advancement and a dedication desire of improving your brain health, there is a treatment that can both rejuvenate your brain and halt future deterioration. There is a way to safely and effectively regenerate the brain, so you no longer need to be at the mercy your most important organ as it experiences deterioration.

There is nothing more gratifying for me than to work with patients who can turn their lives around through the treatment we can offer. I certainly would not be able to do this work alone, were I not surrounded by some of the most inspiring colleagues I've ever met. The task we have set for ourselves, to create a healing environment that is founded on principles of collaboration and optimal integration that give our patients new leases on life, is not a simple one. Only through the fusion of brilliant hearts and minds, from all different backgrounds who share in our mission, is it possible to strive toward providing patients with a better quality of life than what they can currently imagine. Our team wouldn't have been created if it weren't for our patients, people like you who have their hearts set on living the best life available to them.

At their very core, the founding principles of our procedures are based on enhancing brain functions safely and effectively. We aim to give you a healthy brain and body that will not only improve your present quality of life but also can do so right into your later years. I would not attach myself to any procedure that would put anyone at risk or cause harm. As a result, we've learned some novel approaches to treating a brain without compromising on anyone's safety.

Optimal healthcare can only be brought about through teamwork. We combine theory and practice, gathered worldwide, to ensure your treatment is based on the best knowledge possible. This integrative approach differentiates us from other medical practices. By looking at each client from a holistic base, we can provide comprehensive, in-depth treatment.

Aging as the Biggest Medical Complication on the Planet

At East West Clinic, the very core of our mission is the extension of your youth, so that you can thrive in a body that serves you for as long as you need it to. This does not only mean sporting a complexion so youthful that other people think you are lying when you reveal your real age. The cosmetic aspect is part of our work, but it is a happy by-product of our true goal, which is for you to feel like you possess a body and brain that is improving with age. Through this process, we hope to ensure that your days on this planet are spent feeling invigorated by life, rather than eroded by it. For us to do this, we put at the forefront the greatest medical complication on the planet today: aging.

Now, some of you may laugh at this point. "What do you mean? Everyone gets old! Everyone will deteriorate as they move toward death. It's part of life."

It is certain that at some point, you will leave this planet. What is not true is that you must leave this planet in a body that is deteriorating, or with a mind that no longer serves you. It's also not true that we do not have the technology for a person to live (happily) into ripe old age.

My primary wish is for my patients to live a long life. There is so much wonder to experience on this planet. I would like to offer people the gift of time to discover as much as they can while they are here. It is almost impossible to admire the many awe-inspiring marvels of this earth when you are suffering from feeling pain, or the slow erosion of your mind, or the consistent reminder from brain and body that your best days are behind you. My goal is to shift that dynamic for our patients, so that they feel rejuvenated, hopeful, and energized.

If you have read my previous book, **_Your Health Transformation_**, you may have noticed this quote in the acknowledgments:

"I'm so grateful for all the patients who have taught me more than all the universities ever could."

My appreciation and admiration for those brave people who have gone on the journey with me to achieve their health and wellness goals cannot be understated. They have the wisdom to acknowledge that they are not in the place they feel like they should be. The real heroes of our clinic are the patients who are willing to say, "I know that life has more to offer than what I am currently experiencing." For those of you I have already worked with, I say, "Thank you. "To those I have yet to meet, I show my appreciation in advance.

I grow so attached to my patients as I navigate this path with them. One of the saddest days of my life was when one of my favorite patients passed away in her nineties. Her family was very grateful for all of her added years. She managed to live far beyond the point when doctors had told her she would. Still, it was incredibly hard to see her go. I find comfort in the fact that because of the work we do, she was able to see the smiles on her children's faces many more times than she or her family had initially thought possible. She was able to attend the graduation of her grandchild and the wedding of her grand-niece. She got to see the Grand Canyon, a dream of hers since childhood. She saw more springs where blossoms popped out from the cold to delight her, and more winters to cuddle up next to a fire with her dog on her lap. These moments are priceless. If we can open the opportunity for our patients to experience more love, more vitality, and more irreplaceable moments with their loved ones, we have done our job. I am hoping that we can do this for you.

Imagine Your Death (It Will Be Fun, I Promise!)

Right now, imagine that you could choose the age at which you stop living. (For this exercise, you have complete control. It's all up to you.) For this moment, you are allowed to decide: Imagine how you would feel at this age, the energy that you would have, and how you would be living your life. Now get a pen and paper. I challenge you to write down the age that you have decided on, 85 or 90, or whatever number sounds like a good age to you.

Now picture yourself at the age you have written down. Imagine that you have all the resources you could want. You have a support structure, great friends, and family around you. Financially, you are comfortable; maybe you have a little spare money to play around with. You have a purpose. Life feels meaningful.

If all these conditions were met, if you truly felt content and purposeful, would you still want to die at the age of 85 or 90, or whatever number is written on your piece of paper? Picture yourself as very healthy at that age, not plagued by ailments that put you in constant pain or doing battle with a mind that frustrates you at every turn. From this perspective, choose a new age. Write it down. I can almost guarantee you that this second number will be larger than the first.

It may be hard to fathom, but we're moving toward an era when we may be able to determine the age at which we die. Allow me to take you on a journey through some recent discoveries that have groundbreaking ramifications for the way in which we live our lives. This research shakes the foundation of many approaches to health and wellness.

The Youth Extender

One of my mentors is a profoundly inspirational person by the name of Dan Sullivan, the Strategic Coach. He has a practice called The Lifetime Extender. Dan's goal is to live to be 156 years old. With Dan's help, I was able to push my goal out almost 100 years beyond what I had initially imagined.

Yes, you read that correctly:

Dan Sullivan's goal is to live to be 156 years old.

I can hear the responses twittering in your minds. I am sure some of you are saying,

"That's ludicrous! How could anyone ever set that as a goal? It's not possible."

My response is that I wish you could meet Dan Sullivan. He's a bright 74-year-old man. He burns 1,000 calories every day before breakfast. I am privileged to go and spend time with him in Toronto every three months, and every three months he looks more fit than my last visit. If anything, it looks like he is aging backwards.

Do you know what witnessing Dan's determination has done for me? It has given me an epiphany that I would like to share with you. When I see Dan, I think," If you want to live to be 156 years old, you can't have wishful thinking, you've got to have a plan."

Dan Sullivan is an active player in his health. He does not take the back seat and hope for the best. He has 'agency,' the ability to act independently. He is engaged. Dan gets his lab work results reviewed frequently. He is aware of the role played by his genetics in his overall wellness. From a knowledge basis, he ensures that his gut health is at its optimal peak. He follows, to a T, a very tight exercise, and nutrition plan. Dan is doing the work.

If you want to meet your wellness goals, you cannot simply go along for the ride. You have to decide that you are willing to work at it, that a fulfilling and long life is worth fighting for. Only then can you shift the boundaries of what you previously thought was possible. The amazing thing is that once you start adopting healthy habits and reaping the benefits, you will not want to turn back to your old ways. Rather, you will look toward the future and see only possibilities.

The Lifetime Extender is not a freebie. You don't get coupons with this deal. You have to put in the work. You are a key player in the decisions you make and the habits you form. And if you are willing to bring yourself to the party, I can promise that you will not look back.

Aging is the Number One Cause of Death

At this moment, the verified oldest person in the world was a woman from France called Jeanne Louise Calment. She died at age 122 and a half. Can you imagine all the history that Jeanne Calment had lived to witness? She sold pencils and canvases to Vincent van Gogh when she was 14 years old. I wonder if she knew at that point that she had more than 100 years left on the planet.

By looking at the story of either Dan Sullivan or Jeanne Calment, I'm sure we can agree that the potential to prolong the human aging process is something a few people have been able to invite into their lives in various ways. On the flip side, we cannot deny what these and many other stories illustrate for us:

Aging is the number one cause of death.

This presents us with a choice. Do we give in to that fact, or do we do what we can to prolong our lives by staving off the aging process?

I hope that we can walk together to find new approaches to keeping aging at bay long enough to make us feel that we have fulfilled our purpose on this planet. With the new methodologies at our disposal, I would like to propose that, if we are willing to do the work and engage with practices that have been discovered for our benefit, we can slow down the aging process; in many cases, we may be able to reverse it.

But before we go any further, let's have a look at the actual nature of aging.

Aging: Degeneration or Poor Regeneration

The definition of aging is poor regeneration, or the degeneration, of organs and tissues. It is an unfortunate matter of fact that right now, we are losing cells. Perhaps more distressing is that more of our cells die than can be replenished. The process of aging can be defined as this process: losing more cells than we can generate.

Aging is a process that takes place on a cellular level. It follows that if we ask the question, "How can we enhance our health;" the answer must be found within our cellular processes. As much as we would like to think of ourselves as very important, we are essentially the combination of a bunch of cells and bacteria that happen to communicate very well with each other. That combination gives us this thing we call a physical body. What a bizarre miracle our bodies are.

As I have mentioned, aging is the leading cause of death. Let's look at the statistics; as of 2011, 151,600 people die every day[1]. 100,000 of those people die from aging. This is a phenomenal percentage. Our task is not only to see how many of these deaths can be prolonged, but also how the quality improves the lives of those who achieve this longevity.

Next comes the big question: "How can we delay aging?" The answer lies with the very thing we lose as we get older: our cells.

Think about this. You and I are losing over 300 million cells per minute. It is hard to imagine that while you sit, reading this book, you are currently going through a cell degeneration process. If aging is caused by degeneration or the poor regeneration of cells, the way to prolong it is to find ways to repopulate those cells.

The reality is that we wouldn't exist without cells to make up our bodies. If we allow our cells to continue dying in this manner, without attempting to repopulate them, we are moving closer and closer toward our deaths.

----

[1]http://www.ecology.com/birth-death-rates/

Stem Cells in a Newborn

At East West Health, our passion lies in an integrative approach to wellness. We have put much time and many resources into discovering what we can do to stave off the aging process and repopulate our cells. We've found stem cells at the core of the solution. Quite simply, stem cells can replenish cells and prevent cellular death.

You may be wondering, "What exactly is a stem cell?" Think of stem cells as the master cells in your body. These stem cells influence all the basic processes that occur within you. Stem cells repopulate your skin as your skin cells die off and allow for the regeneration of your liver. They oversee the regrowth of your hair follicles, so you get new hair that grows every six months. Perhaps you are aware that every single cell in your liver is repopulated and replenished every three to five days, and your intestines are regenerated every three to five days. Even your brain cells are constantly dying and replenishing every seven to nine days. Your stomach is repopulated every two to three days. Your body is a hard-working regeneration machine—and the workers in this factory are stem cells. If we didn't have stem cells, the degeneration that causes aging would set in much more quickly.

You have a range of different types of stem cells circulating throughout your body, all serving various functions. Hematopoietic or blood stem cells are a collection of immature stem cells[2] found in the peripheral blood and bone marrow. Another type is the mesenchymal stem cells, or MSC[3]. These exist in every artery in your body. The healthier is your blood circulation, the greater the population of these MSCs in your body.

Stem cells may not be that unfamiliar; you may have had degeneration in your knees, for example. A common treatment is to use stem cells to regrow that cartilage. Stem cells have been used for a while to regrow damaged tendons or ligaments. The next obvious step is to look at stem cells as a means of regenerating the brain.

---

[2] https://www.cancer.gov/publications/dictionaries/cancer-terms/def/hematopoietic-stem-cell
[3] https://www.eurostemcell.org/mesenchymal-stem-cells-other-bone-marrow-stem-cells

As we have discussed, the main cause of aging is not having high enough stem cell turnover to repopulate those damaged in your body. Our stem cells do two things as we age. First, the number of stem cells released will decrease as we get older. Second, the stem cells we produce are not as robust as they once were. They are no longer capable of differentiation.

If you observe a stem cell from a newborn baby in a petri dish for 24 hours, you will see it doubling every 24 hours. After 30 days, you'll have a billion new stem cells. This is called 'exponential growth.' The way stem cells operate is truly remarkable. Before a stem cell specializes to fit its designated purpose, it will differentiate and create another stem cell. For example, before an eye cell becomes an eye cell, it creates more of itself, allowing for extraordinary growth.

Stem cells create an abundance of themselves. Each stem cell leaves behind a master cell as a means of repopulating that particular stem cell when it dies, almost like a self-fulfilling insurance policy.

STEM CELL

Brain
Neuron
Intestines
Enterocytes
Hepatocytes
Osteocyte
Bone
Cardiac cells
Heart
Liver

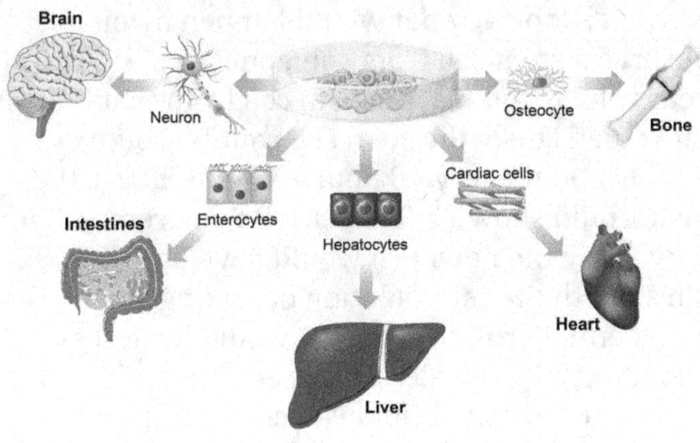

Stem Cells as We Age

Now let's look at what would happen if you observe a stem cell from someone aged 35 or 40 years old. If you place a stem cell from that body into a petri dish, the stem cell counts would double about every 48 hours. After 30 days, the dish would show 32,000 cells. Do you remember how many the newborn would have had after 30 days? With the repopulation occurring at an exponential growth rate, you would have seen about one billion cells. At this age, the repopulation rate is not even close to the number created by a newborn. Now if the stem cell was put into a petri dish from someone aged 65, the number of cells would double every 60 hours. After 30 days, there would only be about 200 cells in that petri dish.

The real goal in combating aging and extending your youth can be achieved through the repopulation of stem cells.

As mentioned previously, up to a certain point of aging, a stem cell can differentiate and populate all the major organs and tissues in your body. Our bodies are made up of a range of different types of cells. Osteocytes are the cells necessary to make up your bones. Cardiac cells are for your heart, hepatocytes are for your liver, enterocytes are for your intestines, and neurons are for your brain. If you have a sufficient quantity of stem cells repopulating all these new tissues, you will be able to stay healthy.

Now for the bad news. Through the aging process, regeneration and repopulation processes become less and less efficient. The rate at which our stem cells double will drop substantially as we get older, but also, the rate of release of our stem cells will decline significantly. By the time you reach the age of 34, the rate at which stem cells are released will be cut in half.

These stem cells are called pericytes[4]—not parasites wanting to suck your blood, but pericytes that are there to help it flow. Pericytes sit on top of the blood vessels. Whenever there is bodily damage such as a loss of blood circulation, a heart attack, or injury to the ischemic tissue[5] which restricts the blood supply to tissues in the body, these pericytes peel off the blood vessels

---

[4]https://www.ncbi.nlm.nih.gov/pmc/articles/PMC4759679/
[5]https://www.ncbi.nlm.nih.gov/pmc/articles/PMC2032306/

and become stem cells. Think of them as on-call backup cells, waiting for us to need them. As we age, their rate of release is cut in half.

Let's think of this regarding our life experience. Think about how quickly you healed from a wound as a baby. You crawled right into objects that would not move out of your way. You cried. Your mom rushed to your aid to see a bleeding gash on your knee. Do you remember what happened to that injury? Well, it wouldn't be surprising if you had completely forgotten it, because there was virtually no scarring to remind you.

At the age of 50, getting a cut may be a little more memorable. It will leave a mark. It takes at least twice the amount of time to heal a cut at age 50, versus as a newborn, because our stem cell release rate drops by 50%. By the age of 65, the stem cell release rate drops by 90%. Not only is the quantity of stem cells diminishing, but also the quality of them. The stem cell's ability to operate productively in your body will diminish by almost 90% by the time you are 65 or older. Think about it. At the age of 65, about 10% of your adult stem cells are circulating in your blood.

Time to Replenish

Through careful analysis, we at East West Health have concluded that the best way to stave off aging and improve our longevity is to increase the amount of our healthy stem cell reserves. What is so groundbreaking about our research is that this process not only pertains to your body from the neck down, now it can also be applied to your brain.

So how can we work at replenishing the stem cells in our brain? I'm going to share a study that shows the level of importance of this research and continue on how we will be able to achieve this for you.

If your childhood was anything like mine, I'm sure you were told countless times, "That [activity, from video games to bungee jumping] will kill your brain cells." I certainly remember being exposed to a specific kind of lacquer paint while building a skateboard ramp, and one of my friends saying, "Man, those fumes are going to kill your brain cells, and once the brain cells are dead, they're dead. They never come back." That illustrates the narrative that has been so entrenched in us: Once the brain is damaged, it can never be restored.

Now, I will not dispute that irreparable damage to the brain is still the case in some very traumatic instances. However, we are finding now, more than ever, that the brain can indeed replenish itself. These cells can come back to life.

Let's talk about *how* this can happen, because at this point, you may be wondering if I have read too many futuristic sci-fi novels. You want to know the ins and outs, the how, and see the research that backs up this statement.

The Results Are In! (A Look at Hypothalamic Neural Stem Cells)

First of all, let's review the research related to a small region of your brain called the hypothalamus[6]. The hypothalamus is part of what regulates all your endocrine functions. A team of age extension researchers[7] conducted experiments on mice to examine the neural stem cells[8] that exist around the hypothalamus. The hypothalamus lies right at the base of your brain. These age extension researchers found that the stem cells in the hypothalamus declined sharply

---

[6]https://www.healthline.com/human-body-maps/hypothalamus
[7]https://www.theguardian.com/science/2017/jul/26/stem-cell-brain-implants-could-slow-ageing-and-extend-life-study-shows
[8]https://www.ncbi.nlm.nih.gov/pmc/articles/PMC3343380/

in mice around the age of 10 months. That's a few months before the onset of clear aging symptoms. By the age of two years, most mice don't have any hypothalamus stem cells left. They're gone. The research team wondered, "Would these mice age faster if these stem cells were gone?"

They wanted to examine whether or not their hypothesis could be true. The next question they asked was, "Do any of these hypothalamic neural stem cells do anything to cause aging in these mice?"

After targeting the brain cells in these otherwise healthy mice with viruses, to selectively destroy the hypothalamic neural stem cells, the researchers found that the results quickened the aging process. These mice had accelerated memory problems and weakened muscles. Their coordination declined. Their sensorimotor system essentially started to shut down, like with aging humans who start walking in a shuffle and lose our coordination and balance. It did not stop there. The mice whose hypothalamic neural stem cells were destroyed also died sooner.

The researchers found their hypothesis to be correct: hypothalamic neural stem cells do influence aging. Their research did not end there. Now they wanted to see what would happen if they replenished the brain with healthy stem cells. Amazingly, they found that the aging pattern was reversed.

The team concluded, "Our research shows that the number of hypothalamic neural stem cells naturally declines over the life of an animal. This decline accelerates aging. We also found that the effects of this loss are not irreversible. By replenishing these stem cells, or the molecules they produce, it's possible to slow and even reverse various aspects of aging throughout the body."[9]

Truly, this is a definitive discovery of our time. Imagine the possibilities of restoring the health of your brain. What if we can get you comfortable with the possibility of extending your life? Think of all the diagnoses you could receive for neurodegenerative issues: Alzheimer's, dementia, Parkinson's, ALS, and so on. Now imagine that you could regenerate some of those damaged systems and tissues in your brain. Isn't that the most life-changing discovery you have ever encountered?

---

[9]Nature.com (2017)
https://www.nature.com/articles/nature23282

A Healing, Hopeful, Helpful Brain

Now what if you have already reached ripe old age, but you are still healthy and mentally fit? Wouldn't you want to live longer, if you had financial resources, great relationships, and purpose? Remember when I asked you to think about that age that you want to live to. What if we crafted a plan together to help you reach the age that you want to live?

Our goal would be to increase your youthfulness with stem cell health in a collaborative way. Keeping your stems cells healthy comes down to living a healthy life. A body's health is reliant on the foods you eat, the thoughts you think, the amount of toxins exposure you receive, and any radioactivity exposure in your environment. All of these factors influence your body's ability to release stem cells, and ultimately to heal itself.

We've seen that stem cells can perform all sorts of miracles in our bodies, such as regenerated knees. Thousands of knees regenerate and become younger as a result of stem cell procedures. We've seen it in hips, spines, and shoulders. Now it is time to turn to the brain.

I must ask you this question: What is the worst part of poor brain health? Is it what we so affectionately call 'brain fog'? Is it tiredness? Is it the embarrassment of being unable to remember somebody's name? How does having a brain that does not perform well, or as well as you would like, affect your relationships and your ability to work, learn, and enjoy life?

The health of the brain is not something I study because it is my job. This issue has had a very real impact in my own life. My grandmother was a phenomenal entrepreneur. She was incredibly charismatic and extremely bright. She ended up with Alzheimer's. Toward the end of my teen years, I remember getting extra birthday cards in the mail. At first, this seemed quirky and endearing. It did not stay that way. I noticed when my grandmother started calling me by my cousin's name. This was so uncharacteristic of a woman who had always been in such control. Quite soon after this, she was diagnosed with Alzheimer's. My last memories of my grandmother are of someone who was very scared, paranoid, confused, and depressed. I don't want to see anyone else go through that. Now I try to remember my beautiful grandmother at the time before her diagnosis. That was my real grandmother.

How to Fuel and Fix Your Brain

By the time my grandmother died, I was already very interested in understanding the brain. As a result, I've studied it for decades. I read my first book on brain health when I was 13 years old. Over the years, I understood that there are a few key nutrients that help feed the brain, which is very important. But one of the biggest breakthroughs that many researchers are starting to agree on is that the brain not only needs good fuel, but it also needs good thoughts. Our brains are hungry. To stay fit and healthy, our brains crave productive learning patterns, and they need a sufficient amount of healthy stem cells. In what ways can we regenerate and extend the health of the brain, especially for those of you who (like me) may have suffered concussions or had lots of stress in your life? Let's look at how we can regenerate the brain and see if it is possible to start with a clean slate.

The very first thing to look at is how we get the perinatal tissue across the blood-brain barrier.

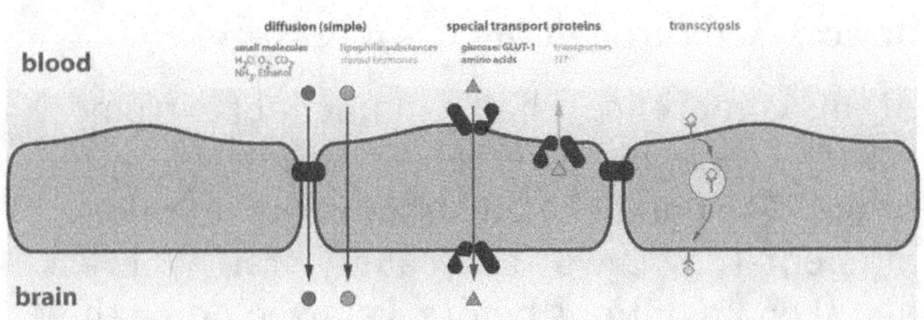

If you look at the image above, you will notice that our brain has a high level of security protecting it. Only very small particles can pass through the blood-brain barrier, and stem cells are too large to receive access.

Historically, the only way that we have been able to breach this barrier, to get stem cells to move through it, is by using a substance called mannitol[10]. This increases the opening of the pores tenfold. It is not always the best method, however, because of the stress placed on the kidneys.

I had the privilege of attending a perinatal stem cell conference. One of the chief researchers there, Arnold Caplan, said the best technique for getting MSCs into the brain is intranasal. He said,

---

[10]https://www.drugbank.ca/drugs/DB00742

"The sensory nerves that allow you to taste and smell are in the sinuses. There is a 'river' that runs across the top of your head and empties into the back of the head. This allows the brain to be accessed through the nasal passages."

At this conference, I had a moment of extreme clarity. I thought, "This is how I can treat my brain!" I've had five concussions, and in this moment, I saw a way to treat my brain where I had seen no options before. I started doing the research.

Intranasal MSC Treatment

Some fascinating research has been done on neonatal brain damage[11]. What researchers have found is that long-term cognitive and sensorimotor improvement can be achieved through intranasal MSC treatments. The treatments can cause an improvement in cognitive function for patients who have suffered a stroke, a brain injury, or a concussion. Treatments have also increased sensorimotor functions, and the results were maintained over time. From this we can deduce that the treatment is very safe.

Why would we want to use the sinuses, as is done with intranasal MSC treatments? First of all, there are no needles or injections, so it's not necessary to perforate any part of your body. Secondly, the human body has provided us with

---

[11]https://www.ncbi.nlm.nih.gov/pubmed/22430383

an accessible opening, a portal to your brain. At this point in your sinus passages, there is your olfactory bulb, which contains nerves. Your hypothalamus is right there in that area, as are the pituitary and pineal glands. Researchers from the Experimental Animal Committee Utrecht (supported by the European Union) have found that these stem cells can migrate throughout the brain[12] in a very short period.

Breaching the blood-brain barrier has been a big issue in the past, raising many questions. For some sample questions, "How can we get enough of these MSCs into the area to signal and create a change in the brain? How can we calm down the brain inflammation?" An inflamed brain can create a loss of your body's regenerative properties, and the release rate of stem cells.

One of the top researchers in this area is a doctor named Dr. William Frey[13], a senior director of neuroscience research at Regions Hospital in Saint Paul, Minnesota. He is one of the top researchers who discovered the intranasal method used for bypassing the blood-brain barrier. Intranasal stem cell and T cell delivery have been validated in animals for the treatment of MS, Parkinson's, stroke, brain tumors, spinal

---

[12]http://journals.plos.org/plosone/article?id=10.1371/journal.pone.0051253
[13]http://www.neuroscience.umn.edu/people/william-h-frey-ii-phd

cord injuries, and other brain disorders. This work was published in Neurology Reviews[14] in April of 2016.

Through collaboration with researchers in Germany, he discovered that intranasal MSC treatments can treat Parkinson's disease, Alzheimer's, and cognitive decline [15]very successfully, as a result of stem cells' ability to bypass the blood-brain barrier and reach the brain. This technique is being investigated in various disorders. While most of the studies have been done on animal models exclusively, investigation into the treatment of Alzheimer's disease has also been done in humans.

Dr. Frey also discovered is that MSCs are not the only aids in the treatment of cognitive disorders. Essentially, stem cells are not doing the work alone. In the perinatal tissue, stem cells are a minor component. Other important components are the cytokines—the growth factors, signaling properties, and paracrine functions of the other cells that exist in this tissue. After treatment, Dr. Frey noticed that the pro-inflammatory cytokines diminished. As a result, the inflammatory brain diseases retreat to normal levels.

---

[14]https://www.mdedge.com/neurologyreviews/article/106892/a lzheimers-cognition/intranasal-drug-delivery-bypasses-blood-brain
[15]http://www.cellr4.org/article/1646

Through the intranasal method of delivery, within a matter of minutes, it has reached the brain and spinal cord. In humans, researchers found that the intranasal neuropeptides reached the cerebral spinal fluid in 10 minutes. The study showed highly significant improvement compared with a placebo treatment in motor function or movement.

What does this mean for you? If you have any neurologically related issues, not merely cognitive decline as a result of aging, this might be a possible treatment for you.

Using Amniotic Tissue

While my mind ticked through all the possible ways to treat or reverse the neurological signs of aging, I thought to myself, "What about using amniotic tissue?" This would mean not only isolating stem cells, but also using the entire tissue including the umbilical cord, the placenta, and the amniotic tissue. I found several things.

One of the studies that I've found for intranasal introduction of amniotic tissue[16] was for MS and macular degeneration. Researchers found that the introduction of this tissue prevents your brain from breaking down and aging. According to this study, the numerous cytokines and growth factors, as presented, suggest possible paracrine activation of multiple intracellular signaling pathways.

---

[16]https://www.ncbi.nlm.nih.gov/pmc/articles/PMC5282572/

You may be asking, "What does this mean, or have to do with the health of my brain?"

As covered previously, you have stem cells for virtually every single tissue in your body. Now, if you can activate your body's stem cells, then your body can start the repopulation process. You have the right cytokines and growth factors; your body needs a little assistance to make your stem cells young again.

I am sure you have had the experience of looking at two people of the same age who seem to be separated by decades. For example, one 50-year-old can look 70, while another 50-year-old can look 30 years old. In the latter example, the 50-year old who looks 30 has done specific things to enhance their stem cell proliferation.

Regarding these growth factors in cytokines, not only do they improve the release rate of your body's stem cells, but they also bring in your body's healing messengers so that your inflammatory messengers calm down. That means many molecules get signaled out from different cells in your body to promote better tissue regeneration.

Isn't this phenomenal? Intranasally-delivered amniotic tissue suppresses inflammation. Research has shown that it prevents neural damage and preserves neurologic function in the experimental autoimmune encephalomyelitis animal model of multiple sclerosis.[17] This amniotic tissue contains a high number of cytokines and growth factors. As it worked with MS, it also worked in preventing vision loss.

So how does this umbilical and amniotic tissue function? The very first thing it does is to hone in on sites of inflammation. Once it has found these places, this tissue will regulate the immune responses. It cuts off these inflammatory cytokines, both interleukin six and TNF alpha.

The other vital operation it performs is the regulation of blood vessel growth. This umbilical and amniotic tissue has been proven to have proteins called TIMP2. These proteins stage and promote new blood vessel growth. If you've ever had a concussion, you will know that your brain does not work quite as well as it used to. If you have a neurodegenerative disease like Parkinson's, your dopamine production is low. You need new blood vessels to carry nutrients to that area because Parkinson's disease is a crisis of the mitochondria in the cell. The cells are not receiving energy. That's where some of the tremors can come from.

But the results do not stop there. Amniotic tissue has been shown to reduce scarring. Say, for instance, you have suffered a stroke. Some scar

---

[17]https://www.ncbi.nlm.nih.gov/pubmed/26036872

tissue will get built up in your brain. This umbilical and amniotic tissue can help repair that scarring. This can also be applied to ALS. All of the neurological systems should be firing in synchronicity to prevent premature cell death so that it can repair and regenerate tissue. Isn't it astounding how many uses this treatment can have?

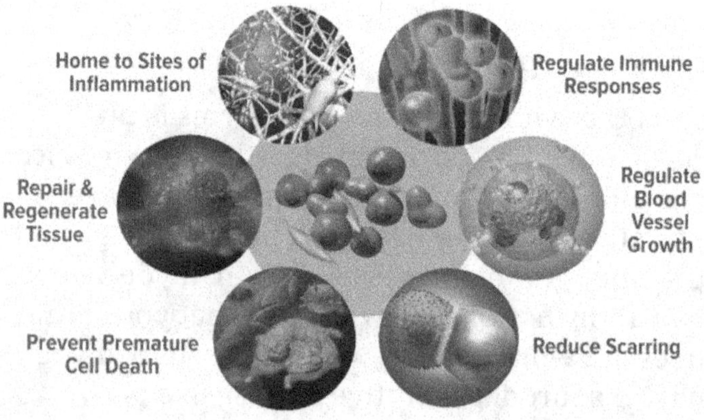

But Is It Safe?

Of course, this is the most important question you can ask when it comes to your precious body and brain. It is also our main concern. From the extensive research we have done on intranasal stem cells and amnion tissue treatments, it seems to be safe. To be clear, the FDA hasn't yet approved this treatment for the prevention or cure of any diseases.

The perinatal tissue used by East West Health falls under Part 1271 of Title 21 of the Code of Federal Regulations and Section 361 of the Public Health Service Act, or the PHS 361 [CFR Part 1271] classification, which means that the tissue cannot be manipulated in any way. We've used amniotic tissue for over 100 years for various conditions very safely, but once the tissue experiences change, so does the safety profile. The FDA oversees all manipulated cellular biologics under section 361 of the PHS Act relating to CFR 1271, and its guidelines. To qualify under section 361, the stem cells would have expanded or changed from their original environment or natural state. This is when stem cells are classified in a similar way to a drug and must undergo more rigorous testing and approval processes through the FDA. I see the unadulterated perinatal tissue, or the CFR 1271/361 tissue allograft, as one of Nature's most potent healing agents available. The fact that it's in a natural biological state allows it to be used for general purposes but not for the prevention or reversal of diseases.

Preliminary research shows that this treatment has broad implications for suppressing inflammation in autoimmune diseases. This is one of the reasons I took the treatment myself. I am living proof that this can work and work safely. It can prevent brain damage in an acute head injury.

In the future, I hope this will become the default first treatment for people who have suffered a concussion. Rather than the current treatment style ("Let's watch it. Go home and see what happens. Don't go to sleep right away."), imagine we could introduce birth tissue intranasally, and in doing so, completely restore the traumatic damage wreaked on the brain.

It is possible that we will be able to calm chronic neurodegenerative diseases such as multiple sclerosis. Research is showing no immune rejection with the introduction of this birth tissue. The birth tissue is in a privileged environment. If you think about, a surrogate mother can carry a baby full-term with no genetic matching at all to the parents and then return the baby, healthy and ready for the world. That describes the incredible safety of this environment.

Right now, in the United States, there are over 4 million births per year. Most of that birth tissue is being discarded. Why is this happening when this tissue possesses massive healing potential? I look at this and think, "The use of this birth tissue is a perfect way of not only decreasing the rate at which you age, but also of improving brain health in people who have degeneration."

The amnion epithelial cells are some of the non-MSC cells that exist in the amniotic tissue. In most cases, there will be about 40 million different types of cells in this amniotic tissue. Some of those will be MSCs, but the majority will be other types of cells. The amnion epithelial cells have been shown to reduce fetal brain injury in response to inflammation. Amnion epithelial cells also modulate immune responses and suppress the inflammatory response in a model of multiple sclerosis. In a model of traumatic brain injury, cell treatment was shown to significantly attenuate axonal regeneration and improve motor impairment. It is simply groundbreaking to have this at our disposal.

But this is the most important part: It has also been found that the intranasal amnion cells are very safe, according to a study published in 2017 from Scientific Report (Intranasal Delivery of a

Novel Amnion Cell Secretome Prevents Neuronal Damage and Preserves Function in a Mouse Multiple Sclerosis Model).[18] According to the study, there are important growth factors in cytokines that stimulate a variety of anti-inflammatory and neuroprotective responses in human cells. These factors may allow cells to respond only to the factors that stimulate receptors and have been upregulated in response to cell stress. I look at this as an amazing means of assistance. Researchers have found that the combination of low concentration of cytokines and growth factors may avoid untoward side effects and may be less likely to stimulate normal levels of receptors in healthy cells. Acute and chronic administration safety studies of amniotic tissue have shown it to be safe and well tolerated.

One of the things found in this report is that the intranasal stem cells were found in virtually every organ system in the body within 24 hours. The lungs, heart, and stomach were the areas receiving the most impact. The report indicated that this delivery mechanism of stem cells could help with the treatment of Parkinson's, strokes, neonatal ischemia, multiple sclerosis, brain tumors, and subarachnoid hemorrhaging.

---

[18]https://www.ncbi.nlm.nih.gov/pmc/articles/PMC5282572/

A Breakthrough Treatment

One of the East West Health stroke patients has undergone the intranasal amniotic tissue procedure. Before the treatment, this patient could only manage single words. She was unable to construct full sentences. After the administration of the amniotic tissue, this patient can now make full sentences. The patient can comprehend the way she is feeling, respond to questions, and participate in her occupational and physical therapy. This patient is meeting goals and exceeding expectations. Without a doubt, her life has been completely transformed by this treatment.

Many people wonder, "Well, where do you get this perinatal tissue? Where does this perinatal tissue come from? What does it look like?"

It may be difficult to envision if you have never been introduced to it before. The first thing you need to know is that it comes from healthy maternal donors.

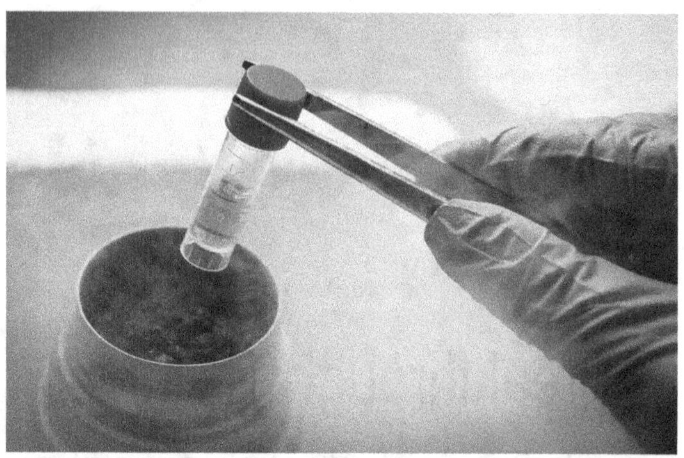

Above is an image of the packaging that the tissue comes in—a vial that gets cryopreserved.

A tissue graft is taken from the placenta. All the birth tissue is taken from the uterus of a donor through a legally performed C-section birth. The mother is pre-screened and pre-tested; any unhealthy mothers are ruled out, or those who have any history showing that they aren't medically fit to donate the tissue. Once the tissue has been returned to the lab and been tested, if any issues are found, then it gets discarded. In all cases, the tissue that is used will come from a healthy mother who is undergoing a C-section birth.

The birth tissue in the cord blood will contain hematopoietic stem cells. These hematopoietic stem cells regulate your immune functions. They create your red blood cells, your white blood cells, and all your platelets.

MSCs will also be found in the tissue. MSCs, as we have discussed before, are mesenchymal stem cells, or 'medicinal signaling cells' as we prefer to call them. These cells can become chondrocytes, osteoblasts, fibroblasts, adipocytes, or glial cells for your brain, skeletal muscles and epithelial cells.

All of these other types of cells exist in the tissue along with growth factors, cytokines, and some of the paracrine secretion cells. So, it is not stem cells we are looking for, but the whole package that the tissue has to offer.

Our samples are locally sourced here in Utah. This tissue is taken from a consenting mother and transported from the hospital, and within 10 minutes, it's taken to the lab. There it gets processed, sterilized, and cryopreserved to protect the cell viabilities.

There's no harm to the baby and no harm to the mother. There is minimal manipulation, meaning these stem cells are not taken out and grown, a procedure which can pose some risks and side effects. Once the tissue has been verified by the FDA, it goes through a period of testing before it is released.

East West Health has used many labs, one of which is the Utah Cord Bank; again, it's locally sourced. The Utah Cord Bank is worth mentioning, as it has been one of the only labs able to produce something called the 'colony-forming unit assay'. Not only has the Utah Cord

Bank shown that their product does have live MSCs, but they've also shown that these cells can form colonies and create new structures.

Note: We use the highest quality and the safest sources that we possibly can.

My Story

This topic is very near and dear to my heart because this treatment has had a profound impact on my life. I always tell people I was the first patient at East West Health to get stem cell therapy in my shoulder. That's my claim to fame, and one that I'm very proud of. It's been over six-and-a-half years since I received my treatment. The result? Well, my shoulder is still doing amazingly.

But my story does not end there. I also treated myself intranasally after I was at that perinatal stem cell conference and heard Arnold Caplan speak about treating brain issues. When I heard Arnold Caplan talk about intranasal as the best application to heal brain function, I said to myself, "I've had a handful of concussions. I want to heal that damaged tissue before it shows up symptomatically as memory loss, Alzheimer's, or dementia."

Not only had I experienced multiple concussions, but also, I had experienced heavy metal exposure and an autoimmune disorder. The first night after my treatment, I had some of the weirdest dreams of my life. It was like my entire brain was organizing and sequencing every thought. I woke up the next day, with some fatigue as the only side effect. But then I noticed that it was almost as if a light had been switched on in my brain. The next night, I continued to have crazy dreams. I woke with a little bit of a headache in certain areas where I've had concussions. I felt pressure there that I typically don't feel.

I believe this pressure to have been the result of the regeneration process, some of those proteins building new vascular responses in my brain. All of my senses seem to have increased their functions. My senses of hearing, sight, taste, and smell had all improved. The biggest victory, of course, was that my memory and cognitive performance felt better. My brain feels quiet, the quietest it's been in years.

The day after the treatment, I did a hard workout. You know what I noticed? My lungs felt better. I've continually noticed that my digestion and sleep have been getting better and better, at least until my wife got a puppy, but that's another story for a different day.

Can We Help You?

I can't make any promises or claims as to whether or not we can help you. The best way to know is to seek out medical advice from your doctor or simply call one of our offices for an evaluation. Once you have decided that you may benefit from this therapy, you might ask, "What does this treatment look like?" It's a simple procedure. There is zero downtime, and no major side effects have been reported in any of the literature or in the patients we've treated.

Who can we help? We can help anyone with neurodegeneration. Of course, that is a very broad scope. Perhaps you are simply looking to improve your brain health. This could be a very viable solution for you. Maybe you are looking for help with cognitive performance. Perhaps you've started to notice, "I'm not quite as sharp as I used to be." This might be the very thing you have been looking for.

Give us a call to find out if you're a good candidate for this treatment. You can find our phone number at **www.acueastwest.com**. Give us a call at our Salt Lake, Saint George, Park City, or Pleasant Grove offices, and we will route you to the closest clinic.

We look forward to talking to you about this. It's something that has intrigued me my whole life. I have seen how it can alleviate pain and transform and extend people's lives. I've had over eight different stem cell treatments. The intranasal was by far the most mind-expanding and enriching treatment that I've had of all eight. Getting rid of pain was huge, but feeling my brain turn on again has been phenomenal. Seeing some of the early results in our patients has been very encouraging. Being a part of this life-changing research has truly changed my perspective on what is possible. I hope it can do the same for you.

If you have any family, friends or loved ones who needs help, then send them our way. We don't have to put up with suffering. We don't have to give in to the dictates of the aging process. Help has arrived. We want you to live a life that is long, beautiful and full. This ability is now in our hands.

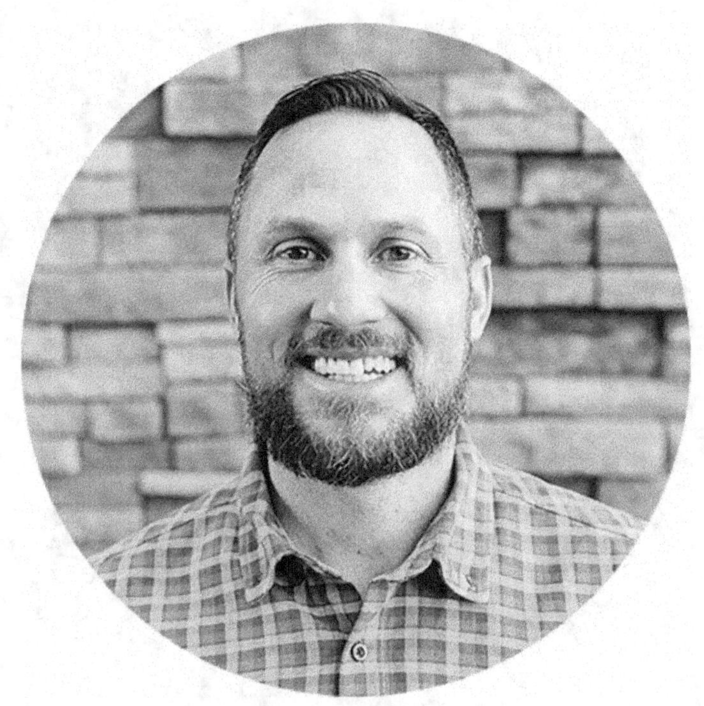

Regan Archibald, Lac, FMP, CSSAc

www.ingramcontent.com/pod-product-compliance
Lightning Source LLC
Chambersburg PA
CBHW061731250726
48657CB00002B/868